LIFE AFTER GESTATIONAL DIABETES

14 WAYS TO REVERSE YOUR RISK OF TYPE 2 DIABETES

BY MATHEA FORD, RDN, LD

PURPOSE AND INTRODUCTION

What I have found through the emails and requests of my readers is that it is difficult to find information about a gestational diabetes program that is actionable. I want you to know that is what I intend to provide in all my books. You can take this information from the book and with immediate action you will have a better outcome in your life.

I wrote this module with you in mind: the mom to be with gestational diabetes who does not know where to start or can't seem to get the answers that you need from other sources. This book will provide information that is applicable to a gestational diabetes mom.

Who am I? I am a registered dietitian in the USA who has been working with kidney patients for my entire 15 + years of experience. I was also in your shoes, as a mom to be with gestational diabetes (and now 2 children who are 7 &9) Find all my books on Amazon on my author page: http://www.amazon.com/Mathea-Ford/e/B008E1E7IS/

My goals are simple – to give some answers and to create an understanding of what is typical. In this series for Baby Steps For Gestational Diabetes, I will take you through the different parts of being a woman with gestational diabetes. It will not necessarily be what happens in your case, as everyone is an individual. I may simplify things in an effort to write them so that I feel you can learn the most from the information. This may mean that I don't say the exact things that your doctor would say. If you don't understand, please ask your doctor.

I want you to know, I am not a medical doctor and I am not aware of your particular condition. Information in this book is current as of publication, but may or may not have changed. This book is not meant to substitute for medical treatment for you, your friends, your caregivers, or your family members. You should not base treatment decisions solely on what is contained in this module. Develop your treatment plan with your doctors, nurses and the other medical professionals on your team. I recommend that you double-check any information with your medical team to verify if it applies to you.

In other words, I am not responsible for your medical care. I am providing this module for information and entertainment purposes, not medical diagnoses. Please consult with your doctor about any questions that you have about your particular case.

TABLE OF CONTENTS

INTRODUCTION

Gestational diabetes mellitus (GDM) is a condition that requires treatment and management throughout pregnancy, resulting in increased risks to both a mother and her child. Although gestational diabetes is often resolved after the baby is born, a woman with GDM may be at greater risk of developing type 2 diabetes later. If you had gestational diabetes with your pregnancy, you do not have to fall into the trap of type 2 diabetes, even if you are at an increased risk. Follow these 14 ideas to take control of your health after you have your baby to reverse your risk and to care of yourself.

WAYS TO REVERSE RISK # 1: BREASTFEED

Breastfeeding has been associated with decreased risks of developing type 2 diabetes among women who have been previously diagnosed with gestational diabetes. Breastfeeding may help some mothers to control their weight after giving birth and can have a positive impact on blood glucose levels during the immediate postpartum period. According to the Wisconsin Department of Health Services, women with GDM who breastfeed their infants may reduce their risk of later developing type 2 diabetes by almost 40%.

THE BENEFITS OF BREASTFEEDING

Breastfeeding is a complete form of nutrition for your baby after birth. It can promote bonding between you and your baby because it is a special time of nurturing growth. Breastfeeding provides so many benefits to both mother and baby that the American Academy of Pediatrics recommends breastfeeding babies exclusively for the first six months of life. Even after six months, babies may still continue to breastfeed and gain the benefits of this nutrition.

Immediately after birth, a mother is already producing breast milk to feed to her baby. The early milk is called colostrum, which is thick and comes out in small amounts. While there doesn't seem to be much of it in the beginning, it is this type of milk that is loaded with antibodies that boost your baby's immunity right from the start. After a few days, your body will begin to produce mature milk in larger amounts, and it is this milk that contains important nutrients as well as the right amount of fat and protein that your baby needs.

Beyond providing immune properties and healthy nutrition for your baby, breast milk also benefits your baby in other ways. Babies who breastfeed may be less likely to develop some types of infections later, including ear infections, gastrointestinal issues, asthma, and allergies. Breastfeeding benefits you as a mother as well. Women who breastfeed have a reduced risk of developing ovarian or breast cancer later in their lives. They may also have less stress and may be more likely to lose weight following delivery.

Despite the positive outcomes associated with breastfeeding, it is not always an easy task for everyone. Some women have difficulties with getting started or maintaining a schedule of breastfeeding. After delivery, talk with your nurse or a lactation consultant, who can help you to understand the best positions for holding your baby, how to latch the baby onto your breast, and how often to feed him or her. A lactation consultant can also help you if problems arise that make it difficult to breastfeed. While it is a natural process of feeding, getting started breastfeeding does not always come naturally and easily for everyone, but don't give up without finding help first if you need it.

It is clear that breastfeeding provides many positive benefits, and researchers have found one more advantage of this feeding method: it can help to reduce your risk of developing type 2 diabetes.

How Breastfeeding Can Impact Diabetes

Breastfeeding may help your body to utilize glucose and fat more appropriately, which means you may be less likely to have uncontrolled blood glucose levels later. The process of lactation, during which your body produces breast milk, improves how your body metabolizes glucose. Through this process, your body may use glucose more appropriately, leading to greater control of blood glucose levels. Breastfeeding your baby for longer periods of time lowers your risk of type 2 diabetes even further. Experts are still learning whether the benefits continue to a specific length of time of breastfeeding and whether you get more benefits if you breastfeed exclusively.

In a study by the *American Journal of Medicine*, women who breastfed their children for at least one month had the same risk of developing diabetes later as women who had never given birth at all. Additionally, those who did not breastfeed their babies were more likely to develop type 2 diabetes later than women who exclusively breastfed their babies for at least 1 to 3 months.

Based on these conclusions, it is beneficial for your health and your risk of diabetes if you breastfeed your baby. Although experts recommend a minimum of six months of breastfeeding after delivery, you can still gain the benefits of greater blood glucose control if you breastfeed your baby for even just one month. By taking the time to establish breastfeeding and setting a goal to breastfeed for at least one month, you may find that you already benefit from the process and have an easier time feeding, which could lead to breastfeeding longer than you expected.

WAYS TO REVERSE RISK # 2: MONITOR GLUCOSE LEVELS

The American Diabetes Association recommends an oral glucose tolerance test during the postpartum period for women who had GDM during pregnancy. This test is typically performed the first time at a prenatal checkup between 24 and 28 weeks' gestation. It checks how the body responds to a rapid influx of glucose taken in through a high-glucose drink. For women who develop GDM, this same test should also be done again at a postpartum visit, between 1 and 6 weeks after delivery, to determine if blood sugar levels are normalizing after GDM. Additionally, the oral glucose tolerance test should also be performed at least every three years following delivery.

THE FASTING GLUCOSE TEST

There are several methods of checking your blood glucose levels after you have delivered your baby. Depending on whether you needed to check your glucose levels regularly and take medications with your GDM, you may need to continue monitoring your glucose levels for a little while after delivery. Your health care provider can help you determine how long you will need to continue to monitor your blood glucose.

Although blood glucose testing is very important to ensure that your glucose levels are returning to normal after delivery, not every health care provider offers blood sugar testing in the postpartum period. While it should be known that early testing after delivery can help to keep you on track with understanding your blood sugar patterns and then managing your levels through diet, exercise, or medication, this test is sometimes overlooked by health care providers. If you attend a postpartum check up, you may need to ask for a blood glucose check if your provider does not offer it right away. Ideally, your blood glucose levels should be tested during the initial postpartum period and then again during the 6 to 12 weeks following delivery to ensure that levels are progressing to normal. Further testing may also be necessary until your levels have reached normal limits.

Your health care provider may have her own method of checking your blood sugar levels after delivery. One way is through fasting blood sugar levels, in which your blood glucose levels are checked after you have gone without eating for a period of several hours. Often, you must fast for about eight hours before a fasting blood glucose level is drawn; for many women, the level is checked first thing in the morning before eating breakfast when they haven't eaten all night.

The fasting glucose test checks your blood glucose levels during a time when you have gone without food for long enough that your blood glucose levels should be low. When testing on an empty stomach, your body will not have had recent food intake and digestion to affect your blood sugar levels. If your blood glucose levels are elevated, even though you have not eaten recently, your body might have trouble utilizing glucose in a normal amount of time. Increased levels of glucose in the bloodstream after a fasting period indicate that either the insulin your body produces is not doing its job well enough (or the cells are resistant to what insulin you do produce), or that your body does not create enough insulin to manage what glucose shows up in your bloodstream.

If you have high blood glucose levels after a fasting glucose test, the test will probably be repeated at a later time. Two different occasions of elevated results will require further testing, often through an oral glucose tolerance test. However, if you have significantly elevated levels of blood glucose when testing (typically greater than 126 mg/dl after fasting), your health care provider may decide to treat your blood sugar levels right away before conducting further tests.

THE ORAL GLUCOSE TOLERANCE TEST (OGTT)

Most pregnant women have had an oral glucose tolerance test (OGTT) at some point during pregnancy to rule out or confirm the presence of gestational diabetes. If you were diagnosed with GDM, it may have ultimately been discovered through the OGTT to begin with. Some women with a history of gestational diabetes need an OGTT at an earlier point during subsequent pregnancies because they are at higher risk of developing the condition again.

The OGTT is another method used to determine how the body processes glucose, even after you have delivered your baby. In some cases, a physician may use an OGTT to confirm the presence of diabetes after you have had several elevated results of fasting blood glucose levels. For some health care providers, the OGTT may be the initial form of testing during the 6 to 8 week postpartum period to determine how your blood glucose is changing after delivery.

The oral glucose tolerance test involves consuming a sweetened drink that is high in glucose. It usually contains about 75 g of glucose in one serving. Your blood glucose level is tested before drinking the beverage and then again at one and two-hour intervals to see how your blood sugar levels respond to the rapid influx of glucose. The initial blood glucose level was drawn to determine a baseline for comparison.

If you still have elevated blood glucose levels two hours after drinking the mixture, your health care provider will make a decision about how best to manage this situation, whether it is by administering insulin or taking oral medications. If you have a diagnosis of impaired glucose tolerance or diabetes after you have your baby, it is no longer considered an extension of gestational diabetes, but is now classified as type 2 diabetes.

LIFESTYLE RECOMMENDATIONS

There are many things that you can do to control your blood glucose levels, not only in the postpartum period, but also well beyond your delivery when you are into full-scale parenting mode. If you had gestational diabetes, you are probably familiar with watching what you eat, monitoring your glucose levels, getting enough exercise, and taking medications. Some of these habits do not need to change after delivery. Some women may assume that because they have delivered their babies and they no longer technically have GDM, they can revert back to eating whatever they like and not monitoring their weight or dietary intake much at all. While this is probably possible from a blood glucose standpoint, it may not be the best method of caring for yourself and can cause your blood sugar levels to eventually become abnormal.

One of the best methods of controlling your blood sugar levels after you have delivered the baby is to continue to eat and live as if you still have GDM. Follow dietary plans by restricting too many sugary foods and refined carbohydrates that can wreak havoc on your blood sugar. Instead, maintain the habits you worked so hard to develop while you were pregnant. Even though you needed to watch your diet and activity levels because of GDM during pregnancy, you can still consider those same positive effects on your health, even after the baby is born. Managing your food intake and making healthy choices as though you still have GDM can help you to maintain good health, it can stabilize your blood glucose levels, and can potentially reduce your risk of later developing type 2 diabetes.

WAYS TO REVERSE RISK # 3: CONTROL INSULIN LEVELS

Increased insulin secretion may result in an increased risk of developing diabetes after pregnancy, as elevated levels of insulin may point to a state of prediabetes and decreased insulin sensitivity from the cells. Although insulin levels are not routinely tested as part of the postpartum exam, women can control their levels of insulin production through diet.

THE EFFECT OF INSULIN SECRETION ON BLOOD GLUCOSE

You may have already learned a bit about the effects of insulin in the body if you have gestational diabetes. Insulin is a hormone that is produced by the pancreas. When you eat a meal and your blood glucose levels rise, your body secretes insulin in response to the elevated blood sugar levels. Insulin helps the cells in the body take in excess glucose to be used for energy. When you develop insulin resistance, your body's cells do not respond as well to the effects of insulin and do not take the extra glucose, resulting in decreased energy and increased levels of glucose in the bloodstream.

Insulin plays another important role in relation to weight and fat distribution. Insulin is responsible for regulating fat metabolism, which is partly based on the types of foods that you eat. When your body secretes insulin in response to increased blood glucose levels, this insulin uses the blood glucose to give our cells energy rather than using stored body fat for energy. In other words, if your blood glucose levels become very high, insulin will work on using the glucose already in the blood to give the cells energy, rather than using the stored fat that is available. This makes losing extra body fat very difficult when insulin is constantly working with the excess glucose from food that you eat at each meal.

This is why it is very important to be aware of how insulin works in the body and how it is affected by the foods that you eat. If your diet consists of foods that constantly raise your blood sugar too high, you will have difficulty losing weight because you will not be using extra fat for energy. Weight loss is an important component of controlling diabetes and for reducing your risk of developing type 2 diabetes after having GDM.

How to Control Insulin through Diet

While portion control is important for cutting extra calories out of your diet, if you want to lose weight, you must also learn to eat the right types of foods. Eating a diet that only consists of empty calories through sugar and refined carbohydrates will not help you to get rid of excess fat, even if you eat very small portions of these foods. When your blood sugar levels spike after a high-carbohydrate meal, the body produces extra insulin to manage the situation. Once the cells have gotten their energy from the blood sugar, excess glucose is stored as glycogen in the liver, which can be used for energy later if needed. However, the body can only store so much glycogen. Once there is enough, excess glucose then just gets stored as fat, which can also be used for energy.

When you eat a meal that consists of high levels of carbohydrates, even if you do not have diabetes, your blood sugar rises very rapidly. If insulin is working properly, you feel a rush of energy and motivation because the cells have taken up the excess glucose. After a while, though, you start to feel a let down again because your blood sugar has dropped and you need more to replace it. You may try to make up for the energy by eating more carbohydrate-rich foods to give you energy again. During this process, your body produces large amounts of insulin to make up for the spikes in blood sugar. However, this excess insulin ends up storing more fat and you may feel like you are on a negative cycle of eating and gaining energy, only to crash later and crave more foods again.

You can control insulin secretion through the foods you eat, to avoid being on the negative cycle of back-and-forth cravings and energy, only to have your blood glucose levels drop again. In fact, if you focus on eating a healthy amount of protein, fat, and complex carbohydrates, you can avoid spikes in blood sugar and regulate the amount of insulin you produce. This will help you to have stable blood glucose levels and will change how your body stores fat because you will not be using as much insulin.

What Foods to Eat

It is important to add a blend of different foods to your diet that will keep your blood glucose levels stable and avoid sharp increases followed by rapid drops in glucose levels. Whether you need to lose weight or not, this kind of eating method is important for how you feel overall, it will improve your energy levels by avoiding the rapid influx of sugar followed by a drop in energy levels.

The goal of eating to control insulin secretion is to focus on eating foods that will not cause a rapid spike in blood sugar levels. This may also be called a diabetic diet or diabetic eating plan. You do not have to have diabetes to follow this type of plan. The positive effects of a diabetic diet will work for almost anyone.

A diabetic meal plan involves controlling the types of foods that you eat while maintaining proper portion sizes to avoid excess calories. Almost all foods are made up of proteins, carbohydrates, or fats, or a combination thereof. These food components are broken down differently through digestion, with carbohydrates having the greatest effect on blood sugar. However, protein and fats also affect blood sugar levels, and even if you want to avoid great spikes in blood sugar levels, you should not avoid carbohydrates entirely. What you eat will affect your blood glucose levels, regardless of what food it is; it is finding the right type of food that is important for blood glucose.

You need carbohydrate foods for energy, but choosing the right type of carbohydrates will still give you that energy without causing too great of fluctuation in your blood glucose. Instead of eating "empty" carbohydrate foods that rapidly raise your blood sugar levels (such as white sugar, flour, bread, or sugared cereals), try to substitute foods that are high in fiber and will still give you energy (brown rice, whole wheat bread and pasta, oats, or cereals with high fiber content).

You do not have to completely cut sugar out of your diet, but it should be regulated and only make up a small portion of your daily intake. You can cut back on sugar in a variety of ways, such as through reducing the amount you add through cooking or baking; cutting back on sugary drinks, such as soda or juice, or eating smaller portion sizes for dessert. Additionally, if you do decide to eat a sugary treat, try to incorporate it as part of your regular meal instead of as a snack by itself.

The glycemic index is a measure of how quickly your body converts food into glucose during digestion. When a food has a low glycemic index, it produces glucose more slowly than one with a high glycemic index. Choosing foods that are considered to be low on the glycemic index can prevent great fluctuations in blood glucose and instead allow the body to adjust with a slow and steady rise in blood sugar after a meal.

As an example, you can reduce the amount of foods you eat that have a <u>high glycemic</u> index, some of which include:

- White potatoes, including fries and mashed potatoes
- White bread and pasta, white rice
- Sweetened drinks, candy, and soda
- Snack cakes, cookies, and brownies
- Potato chips
- Beer and hard liquor

Low glycemic foods release blood glucose more slowly and keep your levels stable, which reduces excess insulin release. Try to choose more foods with a low glycemic index to maintain better control of your blood glucose levels. Examples of foods that have a <u>low glycemic</u> index include:

- Vegetables, such as broccoli, cauliflower, radishes, peppers, or asparagus
- Fruits, including apples, pears, peaches, plums, or berries
- Brown rice, whole grains, barley, or oats
- Whole grain cereals and snacks
- Red wine
- Nuts, seeds, beans, and eggs

This method of eating does not have to be classified as a "diabetic diet." You can incorporate this healthy eating method into your daily life and that of your family by making simple changes every day. Once you are in the habit of eating less sugary and processed foods, you may find that eating healthy foods to control your blood sugar is satisfying and tastes great.

WAYS TO REVERSE RISK # 4: INCREASE PHYSICAL ACTIVITY LEVELS

Regular physical activity provides many benefits, including weight loss, improved mental health and positive feelings, and stabilization of blood glucose levels. Regular exercise can also reduce the risk of heart disease that may result as a complication of type 2 diabetes. Engaging in 150 minutes of moderate exercise each week can foster weight loss and improve glycemic control, as well as reduce the overall risk of type 2 diabetes after having GDM.

HOW EXERCISE AFFECTS DIABETES RISK

Regular exercise strengthens the body and the spirit, and it provides positive benefits even if you are just starting out. Because being overweight or obese can significantly impact your odds of developing type 2 diabetes after delivery, weight control is very important. One of the best methods of weight control is through regular exercise. Exercise works to help you lose weight or avoid gaining weight because your body uses calories. Many of the calories that you take in through food are used for energy, but excess calories may be stored as fat. Exercise requires extra levels of energy; it also uses more calories, which leaves fewer calories available to be stored as fat.

Your metabolism is the process of how quickly you burn calories, which has an impact on weight. Some people have a higher level of metabolism and so they burn calories more quickly, while others have slower rates of metabolism and may have a harder time losing weight if they need to. Metabolism can also slow down with such factors as increasing age, heredity, and if you have little muscle mass. Exercise works to increase your muscle mass and can thereby increase your metabolism rate, helping you to burn calories more quickly.

Exercise is also great for strengthening the cardiovascular system. The heart is a muscle that responds to regular intervals of increased activity with use, causing it to become stronger. As your heart muscle strengthens, it is able to pump blood more efficiently, which provides necessary oxygen-rich blood to your tissues. People with uncontrolled diabetes may experience decreases in circulation due to excess glucose in the bloodstream, as well as damage to the blood vessels. Strong blood circulation from a strong heart that pumps blood efficiently can help to offset some of the effects of high blood glucose in the bloodstream.

Finally, increased levels of exercise can help to lower your overall insulin levels. Excess levels of insulin in the body can cause resistance from the cells, and they may be more likely to reject the work of insulin to help them take up excess glucose from the bloodstream. Excess glucose that is not used can also be stored as fat, which contributes to more weight gain. Exercising regularly can help your overall weight goals as well as help you to control your blood glucose levels, which can further decrease your risk of developing type 2 diabetes.

IDEAS FOR EXERCISE AND RECOMMENDATIONS

If you want to start an exercise regimen to boost your health, you have many options for implementing more activity into your lifestyle. The amount of exercise that you need depends somewhat on your age and current level of activity. If you are starting an exercise program but you have not exercised in a while, talk with your doctor about the best method of getting started. In some cases, you may need to slowly increase your activity levels until you reach your goal.

According to the Centers for Disease Control and Prevention (CDC), adults between the ages of 18 and 64 years should get 150 minutes of moderate-intensity exercise each week. This is equal to 2 ½ hours of physical activity that will increase your heart rate and cause you to breathe faster. In addition to this moderate-intensity exercise, the CDC recommends at least two days a week of strength training activities. These are exercises that build muscle and that work all major muscle groups of the body.

Moderate-intensity exercise may also be referred to as aerobic activity. This means that your heart is pumping at a higher rate than when you are resting or even doing everyday activities. You might start sweating or have a little more difficulty talking when you are working out at a moderate-intensity level. To get 150 minutes of this type of exercise each week, you should strive for approximately 30 minutes of activity for five days out of the week. Thirty minutes at a time might sound like a lot of activity, and if you are unaccustomed to exercising at all, this may be a tall order. Break it down into shorter segments: research shows that exercising at a moderate-intensity for 10 minutes at a time will still result in great benefits. If you can, try three 10-minute segments of exercise to reach your 30-minute goal for the day.

There are many different types of activities that count toward moderate-intensity exercise. Some examples include walking, jogging, aerobics, dancing, swimming, biking, or hiking. Some people enjoy team sports such as basketball, football, or soccer; while others enjoy more solitary activities, such as skiing or yoga. There are even some things you can do at home that will contribute toward exercise, including mowing the lawn or gardening.

Working out is not always easy when you are just getting started, especially if you have a newborn to care for as well. You may consider taking the baby with you when you work out, such as by using a jogging stroller or walker on outings or utilizing childcare at a fitness facility. Alternatively, exercise may be a time when you take a break from routines and requirements and do something for yourself. Many people often find that they have trouble getting started exercising, but once they are doing it, they feel great. Whatever your situation, find time to add exercise to your routine, which will help your stress levels, improve your waist line, strengthen your heart, and reduce your risks for diabetes.

Centers for Disease Control and Prevention. (2011). *How much physical activity do adults need?* Retrieved from http://www.cdc.gov/physicalactivity/everyone/guidelines/adults.html#Aerobic

WAYS TO REVERSE RISK # 5: SET A WEIGHT LOSS GOAL

The National Diabetes Education Program (NDEP) recommends that women diagnosed with gestational diabetes should strive to lose weight after giving birth to reduce the risk of type 2 diabetes. The goal for weight loss is to return to pre-pregnancy weight, but this loss should happen over time rather than through drastic calorie reduction. Ultimately, the goal for weight loss should be within six months to one year after delivery.

THE IMPORTANCE OF WEIGHT CONTROL ON DIABETES PREVENTION

Controlling weight is one of the most effective strategies for managing your risk of type 2 diabetes after having GDM. However, this is often easier said than done. It may be very difficult to lose weight after being pregnant, as weight gain is a normal and healthy component of pregnancy to begin with. Additionally, taking steps to make dietary changes and to include exercise into your daily routine may be difficult while trying to simultaneously manage the needs of your baby.

Weight loss does not have to be rapid in order to gain the effects. In fact, rapid weight loss may be counterproductive because if the weight comes off too quickly, you may be less likely to maintain the loss for the long term. Instead, you can make small changes in your lifestyle each day that promote weight management. The goal of weight management for women with GDM is to return to their pre-pregnancy weight within 6 to 12 months after delivery. If returning to pre-pregnancy weight is not an option or you are unable to lose that much weight during this time, a loss of 5 to 7% of your current weight will still provide benefits.

Losing weight and eating healthy foods may be difficult because eating is such an important part of life, both for physical needs as well as social interactions. You can incorporate healthy eating and find foods that you enjoy that will still allow you to eat with pleasure. Make an eating plan that outlines what and how much you will eat each day so that you will have less temptation when you do not know what to eat if you become hungry. If necessary, ask a nurse or dietician for helpful eating plans that can give you energy but help you lose weight.

STRATEGIES FOR WEIGHT LOSS

In addition to increasing activity levels, what and how much you eat are significant components of the weight loss journey. It is helpful if you plan ahead to know what you will eat each day in order to be sure that you are getting enough nutrients for yourself but also fostering weight loss. Overall, you should be taking in fewer calories than you are using through activities in order to lose weight. Some of the following strategies may help as you consider ways to cut back on calories and modify how much you eat each day:

- Instead of three large meals a day, try to eat six smaller meals to space out your food intake throughout the day
- Use smaller sizes of plates so that you do not feel the need to fill up a large dinner plate with each meal
- Slow down when eating and focus on enjoying your food; eating faster may cause you to eat more
- Learn about appropriate portion sizes and stick with them: read food labels to understand what is classified as a serving size as well as how many calories are present in each serving
- Eat when you feel physically hungry, rather than eating because of feeling tired, bored, or because the food is there and it's time to eat
- Focus on taking in between 1500 and 2000 calories each day; if you are breastfeeding, you may need even more calories

What you eat is as important as how much you eat when trying to manage your weight. If you watched your carbohydrate intake and your intake of sugar because you had GDM, it will be beneficial to continue this eating practice after you have the baby instead of reverting back to old habits. If you are new to eating healthy, a few guidelines for what types of foods to eat may be necessary.

1. *Choose whole grains over white flour and starch.* If you can eat at least half of your daily intake of grains with whole grains, you will gain greater benefits of increased fiber and more nutrients. Some types of whole grains to include are brown rice, whole-grain bread, or popcorn.
2. *Take in 1 to 3 cups of whole (or unprocessed) fruits each day.* The amount you need depends if you are breastfeeding your baby. Fruits

are naturally high in vitamins, they taste delicious, and you have a variety of choices, such as strawberries, bananas, kiwi, grapes, apples, oranges, or pears.

3. *Get a variety of vegetables.* Vegetables come in a variety of colors, from orange and green to yellow or purple. Strive to vary the colors of your vegetables and you will get the full benefit of their nutrients with few calories. A range of vegetables to choose from includes lettuce, red or yellow peppers, eggplant, carrots, or broccoli.

4. *Choose low fat when it comes to dairy.* Dairy products are full of calcium but some products may contain extra fat. Pick low-fat yogurt and cheese and look for skim or 1% milk instead of full-fat products.

5. *Opt for lean proteins.* Lean cuts of beef, as well as turkey, chicken, and fish provide for your daily protein needs while offering less fat. You can also take in protein through other sources, such as beans, peanut butter, or seeds.

6. *Choose oils and fats carefully.* Stick with unsaturated fats and try to avoid fats and oils that have saturated fats or trans fats.

There are many small changes you can incorporate into your daily life that will promote weight management. By making a few small changes at a time, you will develop new habits that do not seem so daunting but that are helping you to stay healthy. Losing weight and maintaining a healthy weight will not only help you to feel better, but you will also be able to better manage your blood glucose levels and reduce your risk of developing type 2 diabetes later.

Ways To Reverse Risk # 6: Consider Medications

Although lifestyle modifications can make a significant difference in reducing the risk of developing type 2 diabetes, some women benefit from using oral diabetes medications. A 2008 study from the *Journal of Clinical Endocrinology and Metabolism* showed that women with gestational diabetes reduced their risk of developing type 2 diabetes by 53 percent when they took metformin, a medication often used to treat type 2 diabetes. Metformin is an oral medication that works to control blood glucose levels.

How Oral Medications Affect Glucose and Type 2 Diabetes

Depending on the extent of your gestational diabetes, you may have needed oral medications or even insulin to control your blood glucose levels. Oral medications are often necessary when diet and exercise are not enough to control your diabetes. Oral medications are typically used for people with type 2 diabetes because the condition is caused by insulin resistance. These medications work by lowering your blood sugar levels. If you have very high levels, they may not bring your blood sugar into the normal range, but can at least lower it to some extent. Some people who use oral medications can effectively control their blood glucose levels with one type of medication only; others may need to use more than one type of medication.

Oral medications come in several forms that work in different ways. Some may block how the body digests carbohydrates, which affects how much blood sugar is created after eating. Other types of medications may work by lowering levels of insulin resistance of the cells so that they more readily take up excess glucose for energy and blood glucose levels are normalized.

Additionally, some types of medications work quickly to respond to blood glucose levels, while others are longer acting. Some types last longer than others as well. There are some women who had GDM who find that they need to continue taking oral medications for diabetes because their blood glucose levels do not return to normal levels after having the baby. While this is not always the norm, it is something to consider, particularly if you had difficulty with your blood sugar levels during pregnancy.

Metformin

There is evidence that one specific type of oral medication used for type 2 diabetes is effective against preventing type 2 diabetes later among women who had gestational diabetes during pregnancy. Impaired glucose tolerance is a condition in which your blood glucose levels may be higher than normal but are not classified as being high enough to be considered as a diagnosis for diabetes. Impaired glucose tolerance puts you at risk of developing type 2 diabetes. A study found that women with gestational diabetes who took metformin reduced their chances of developing type 2 diabetes over the course of three years.

Metformin is an oral diabetes medication that is typically used to treat type 2 diabetes. It works by decreasing how much glucose is taken into the bloodstream after eating and it decreases insulin resistance by the body's cells. Metformin is sometimes used with other types of oral diabetes medications or even with insulin to increase its effectiveness.

If you had GDM while pregnant, you should have your blood sugar levels tested after delivery and during a later postpartum check to ensure that your levels are returning to normal. If your health care provider finds that your levels are not within normal limits, you may need to make more intensive lifestyle changes, such as through diet and exercise, in order to control your blood glucose. Continued elevated levels of blood glucose after delivery does not necessarily indicate that you have diabetes. You may be diagnosed with impaired glucose tolerance at first; however, because this condition is a major risk factor for type 2 diabetes later, you will need to carefully follow your blood glucose levels to ensure they are not continuing to creep up to higher levels. Your health care provider may opt for oral medications to keep your blood glucose levels within a normal range and to avoid progression into type 2 diabetes.

WAYS TO REVERSE RISK # 7: ATTEND POSTPARTUM CHECKUPS

Those visits to the OB/GYN do not stop after the baby is born. New mothers will need postpartum visits to the doctor to follow up on weight and blood glucose levels, as well as to determine the amount of healing after delivery. The doctor or midwife may recommend a number of interventions to help with risk factors that could contribute to type 2 diabetes.

WHAT TO EXPECT AT FOLLOW UP VISITS

Follow-up visits are important to ensure that you are healing and staying healthy after you have delivered your baby. These visits are also a time at which your blood glucose levels are checked following GDM to ensure that your levels are returning to normal. It is essential that you make and go to your follow up appointments as ordered by your health care provider so that you can receive continued care after your baby's delivery and to support your overall health.

The first follow-up visit technically occurs in the hospital after you have had your baby but before being dismissed. Your health care provider will visit with you about a number of things to be aware of when you go home with your baby, often including some measures of self-care and watching your blood glucose levels. You will also most likely receive a lot of information from the nursing staff, who can further guide you on adjusting to life at home with a new baby and protecting your health at the same time.

You will also need one or more visits to the health care provider's office for postpartum care. These appointments are necessary to discuss how well you are healing after delivery and if you are feeling emotionally well. Not only are these visits important for ensuring that your blood sugar is under control and that you do not continue to have insulin resistance, but you may have other tests as well. These tests and assessments are important to protect you against complications such as infection or the development of certain chronic diseases, including hypertension.

The postpartum check up is an important time to discuss any issues that you might be having that can affect your health and well being. For instance, some women continue to have pain after delivery, which needs to be addressed at the postpartum visit. Your health care provider may discuss any number of topics with you, depending on your current state of health, including weight control, exercise, glucose control, high blood pressure levels, sexual health, or breastfeeding concerns. You will probably have an appointment scheduled for your first postpartum visit by the time you are ready to take your baby home after delivery. If you develop complications or you otherwise have concerns before your first visit is scheduled, however, do not wait until your appointed time. Instead, call your doctor's office and share your concerns. You may need to be seen before your scheduled appointment.

SOME TESTS THAT MIGHT BE ORDERED FOR DIABETES PREVENTION

If you are a new parent, you may be unsure of what to expect at your postpartum visits. On the other hand, if you have had children before, a routine postpartum visit might be second nature to you. Here are some of the things you can expect at a postpartum visit after you have had your baby:

- A check of your vital signs, including your heart rate, respirations, temperature, and blood pressure
- A check of your height and weight
- A pelvic exam to ensure that your body is healing appropriately
- An abdominal exam if you have had a cesarean section, to ensure that your incision and the surrounding tissues are healing appropriately
- Laboratory tests, such as a glucose test or a blood level to test for anemia
- Immunizations, if you need to catch up with certain vaccines

While not directly related to your blood glucose in all assessments, these tasks are an important part of maintaining your health. Through these assessments and tests, your health care provider can determine if you are remaining healthy and can direct your efforts toward how to care for yourself in certain areas.

This is also a time to discuss any concerns that you may have about your health. Do not hesitate to bring up these important matters. If you are not feeling well or you feel that something is just plain wrong, talk to your health care provider or nurse about the situation. The goal of postpartum visits is to ensure that your health needs are met after the baby arrives. If something is bothering you, this is a time to bring it up.

WAYS TO REVERSE RISK # 8: MONITOR CHOLESTEROL LEVELS

While cholesterol is often viewed as affecting the body in a negative way, your body needs some cholesterol to stay healthy. In fact, much of the cholesterol that your body needs it also produces through the liver. Cholesterol is used to form the protective covering over the nerves and makes up part of the cell membranes. Extra cholesterol also enters the body through the diet when you eat certain foods.

CHOLESTEROL AND ITS EFFECTS ON THE BODY

Cholesterol is a type of fat that is normally found in animal-based foods such as meat and eggs. Cholesterol molecules connect to protein in the bloodstream to form lipoproteins, and cholesterol types are typically referred to as low-density lipoproteins (LDL) or high-density lipoproteins (HDL). The cholesterol known as LDL has also been called "bad" cholesterol because excess amounts contribute to heart disease. Increased LDL cholesterol can build up in the arteries and form plaque deposits that result in hardening of the arteries, also called atherosclerosis. This condition reduces blood flow to important organs, including the heart and the brain.

High-density lipoproteins may also be referred to as "good" cholesterol because they positively impact the body. HDL cholesterol gets rids of extra amounts of LDL cholesterol by finding it and taking it to the liver where it can be reused. HDL cholesterol may also reduce the amount of plaque that builds up in the arteries during atherosclerosis, further reducing its effects.

Triglycerides are another form of fat found in the bloodstream. When combined with high levels of LDL cholesterol, triglycerides contribute to atherosclerosis and heart disease. The body changes extra calories and sugar into triglycerides when you take in too much through your diet.

MAINTAINING NORMAL CHOLESTEROL LEVELS

Experts have set recommendations for what levels are considered normal for cholesterol numbers. If you have never had your cholesterol level checked or it's been a while since you found out your results, you may want have your levels checked at your next doctor's appointment. Knowing your results can also help you to know if you need to focus your efforts on lowering your numbers or if your healthy habits are keeping your cholesterol levels in the normal range.

According to the American Heart Association, total cholesterol, which consists of your HDL levels, your LDL levels, and part of your triglyceride levels, should remain at or below 200 mg/dl. LDL cholesterol levels should remain below 100 mg/dl and triglyceride levels should ideally be below 100 mg/dl as well. Alternatively, HDL levels should be above 60 mg/dl to better protect you from the effects of heart disease.

You actually do not need to take in any cholesterol through your diet to meet your body's needs, but it is found in many foods and is hard to avoid if you consume foods such as meat, dairy, and eggs. However, there is no cholesterol in plant-based foods such as fruits, vegetables, and whole grains. You can help to control your cholesterol levels by eating more of these types of foods since they will not contribute excess cholesterol to your body.

If you do eat meat, choose products that are low in fat or remove some of the excess fat during preparation and cooking, such as by cutting the skin off of poultry or draining excess fat from ground beef. Choose dairy products that are low in fat as well, such as non-fat yogurt or cheese, and skim milk. Look for foods that contain little or no saturated fats and trans fats.

American Heart Association. (2013). *What your cholesterol levels mean.* Retrieved from
http://www.heart.org/HEARTORG/Conditions/Cholesterol/AboutCholesterol/What-Your-Cholesterol-Levels-Mean_UCM_305562_Article.jsp

WAYS TO REVERSE RISK # 9: RETURN FOR TESTING REGULARLY

Follow-up appointments after GDM are important not only in the postpartum period, but on a continuing basis. Many practitioners will test blood glucose levels during the first 6 to 12 weeks' postpartum, but continued checks of blood glucose levels as well as hemoglobin A1C levels should continue on an annual basis either with your regular physician or gynecologist.

THE IMPORTANCE OF CONTINUED GLUCOSE MONITORING

Glucose monitoring is an important part of your postpartum check ups to determine if your blood glucose levels are returning to normal after having gestational diabetes. Many health care providers will perform a check of your blood glucose levels during the immediate postpartum period while you are still in the hospital and then again during at least one of your postpartum checks in the office, typically between 6 and 12 weeks later.

If your blood glucose levels return to normal during the postpartum period, you may feel free and clear. But blood glucose testing should not end entirely. Although you will not need to regularly check your blood glucose levels once they have returned to normal, you should keep an eye on your blood sugar over the long term to ensure that you are not creeping toward diabetes.

Having gestational diabetes during pregnancy puts you at greater risk of diabetes in the future. You may be more likely to develop GDM with future pregnancies and you are also more likely to develop type 2 diabetes later. If you combine these risks with other factors such as your weight and fat distribution (including whether your carry more weight on your hips or your abdomen), hereditary factors, your age, and your activity levels, you may be at great risk of a future diagnosis of diabetes. It is important to check your blood glucose levels periodically and follow up after the postpartum period on an annual basis.

Your health care provider may order a test called the hemoglobin A1C test, which looks at your blood glucose levels over a longer period of time; rather than in a snapshot, such as during a fasting glucose test, or after consuming high glucose content. The hemoglobin A1C is a blood test that checks your red blood cells and can determine if you have had elevated blood sugar levels for the past 2 to 3 months. The red blood cells are responsible for carrying oxygen to the tissues as they travel throughout the bloodstream. Oxygen molecules bind to a small protein found on each red blood cell that is called hemoglobin. Low levels of hemoglobin mean lowered levels of oxygen to the tissues because of decreased oxygen-carrying abilities of the red blood cells.

When your blood glucose levels rise following digestion, the body secretes insulin to get the cells to take up excess glucose from the bloodstream and to use the glucose for energy. Excess glucose from high levels in the bloodstream also attaches itself to the hemoglobin found on the red blood cells and then stays there, traveling throughout circulation for the life of the cell. Each red blood cell has a lifespan of approximately 2 to 3 months, so if glucose particles attached themselves to the hemoglobin of a red blood cell, they would remain attached for the next 2 to 3 months as well. A hemoglobin A1C level tests the amount of glucose that is bound to hemoglobin on the red blood cells. Because of the lifespan of the red blood cell, the results indicate a pattern of how much glucose has attached to the red blood cell over its lifespan, giving clinicians a better idea of how your blood glucose levels have been for the past three months or so.

Hemoglobin A1C results are given as a percentage. A normal or goal hemoglobin A1C level is less than 5.5 to 6%, but many health care providers prefer to have their patients with diabetes keep their A1C levels at a different level, such as 6.5 to 7%. If you had gestational diabetes, your hemoglobin A1C goals may be higher as well.

You can maintain a better understanding of your blood glucose levels over time if you have your hemoglobin A1C levels checked annually by your health care provider. Because this test shows the trends of your glucose results, you can have a good idea of what is going on in your body when you eat meals and learn how your body responds. Additionally, if you have an elevated hemoglobin A1C level, you can take steps to modify your diet and make changes to your lifestyle that can help to control your blood glucose levels and your A1C results may be better the next time. This gives you better control by helping you to manage your blood glucose and keeps you informed. Remaining educated and informed about your health is one of the best defenses against illness and disease.

WAYS TO REVERSE RISK # 10: MANAGE STRESS AND TREAT DEPRESSION

Having a baby, even though usually considered a positive change, can still cause stress for new mothers. Increased stress due to lifestyle changes and infant care can lead some women to feel powerless over managing their health. Additionally, postpartum depression may lead some women to avoid self-care measures, increasing the potential for unhealthy eating habits, decreased activity levels, and weight gain. While it is difficult when feeling stressed and/or depressed after giving birth, providing the right amount of self-care through diet and exercise is essential to support health and prevent diabetes.

MANAGING STRESS

Pregnancy, delivery, and the postpartum period are all stressful events for both your physical and your emotional health. Stress can sneak up on you: you may feel excited about your new child and happy to have visitors but over time, you may feel stress from keeping up with demands for child care, your schedule, and your health. Alternatively, you may feel stress right away if you do not feel well after delivery, or if you or your baby has had complications.

Stress negatively impacts your blood glucose levels and your body overall. Your blood sugar levels increase when you feel stress and if you had gestational diabetes, you may need help continuing to manage your glucose levels if your body does not produce enough or utilize enough insulin to compensate. If you feel continued stress over time, you may have difficulty getting your glucose levels to return to normal. Stress also causes the blood pressure to rise temporarily, which could lead to fluctuations in blood pressure levels. Your body secretes greater levels of stress hormones, which not only contribute to elevated blood sugar levels, but may make you feel other negative symptoms as well. Many people with stress feel more physical pain, such as headaches; sleep problems, or muscle tension. They often feel worried, anxious, irritable, or depressed. These feelings may also lead you to make more unhealthy choices, such as by eating more foods for comfort but that are not healthy.

If you are feeling more stress, there are many steps you can take to help manage your situation, even if you cannot change the circumstances that might be causing the stress. Although you might want to isolate yourself, try to stay active and maintain an exercise regimen. Follow a healthy diet and try to avoid junk food, which can cause a roller coaster effect on your blood sugar levels. Spend some quiet time alone if you can, taking deep breaths and thinking peaceful thoughts. Avoid tobacco or drinking alcohol, as these can adversely affect your health.

Stress management techniques may take some time to learn. Unfortunately, many people who feel stress do not necessarily feel that they have time to stop and take some time for themselves. It is essential, however, to take some of this time for yourself each day to control your stress levels and to prevent fluctuations in blood sugar levels as well as negative health outcomes.

POSTPARTUM DEPRESSION

Some women, despite the excitement and joy that often comes with having a baby, develop postpartum depression. This is not uncommon, based on the fluctuations in hormones that occur after delivery, as well as the ups and downs of keeping a new schedule and caring for a new child. Postpartum depression is not a sign of weakness, nor is it something to be ashamed of. However, if you do develop symptoms of postpartum depression, talk with your health care provider to get help for treating this condition.

It is common to feel a certain amount of letdown after having a baby and "baby blues" occur to some extent in most new mothers. You may feel some sense of sadness or irritability, and these symptoms can occur as mood swings that come on rapidly and unexpectedly. Postpartum depression is more significant and may involve symptoms of the blues as well as difficulty sleeping, changes in appetite, anger, guilty feelings, social isolation, a decreased desire to attach to your child, and thoughts of self harm. It is important that if you have these feelings that you talk with a health care provider right away. Your health care provider can help you in several ways, such as through counseling, medication for depression, or even hormone therapy.

If you had gestational diabetes during pregnancy, you may be more likely to develop postpartum depression. The exact relationship between these two conditions is still unknown, but they may be related because of hormone changes associated with blood glucose fluctuations of diabetes.

Post partum blues and depression also place you at greater risk of loss of blood glucose control because the feelings and lack of motivation that often comes with these situations may make it more difficult to control your diet and to monitor your blood glucose levels. You may decide to eat more unhealthy foods as a result of your feelings or alternatively, you may feel as if you don't have much of an appetite at all. Both situations can negatively impact your blood glucose levels. Additionally, it takes time and motivation to check your glucose levels, take medications, watch your diet, and generally just care for yourself after delivery. If you are suffering from depression, you may have less motivation for these tasks, which can cause an increased risk in blood glucose levels and poor health.

Don't wait to talk with someone if you think you have postpartum depression. Starting treatment for this situation can quickly help you get back on track and you can better take care of yourself and your baby.

WAYS TO REVERSE RISK # 11: ALLOW FOR HEALING

The birth of a baby requires a time of healing and repair for the body. Postpartum mothers need to take time to heal and rest after birth, regardless of the type of delivery. Self care after delivery will minimize the risk of infection, which places great stress on the body. Stress hormones can cause changes in blood glucose levels, which can make blood sugar levels more difficult to maintain.

THE EFFECTS OF HEALING AFTER DELIVERY

Pregnancy and childbirth will cause changes in your body, which will take some time to get used to. Some of these changes will be permanent, while others will require you to manage them through rest and time to get back into a routine again. The initial days and weeks after you have a baby should be a time of rest to allow your body to heal. This can be incredibly difficult when you have to take care of a new baby, but taking some time for your own self-care is extremely important to avoid complications that occur from poor healing.

Take the time to rest as much as you can, this will not only allow your body to heal from delivery, but will provide emotional recovery as well. A baby's birth is a whirlwind of activity, followed by a number of different emotions, feelings, and hormone changes that can leave you feeling happy and excited one minute and tearful or angry the next. Take time to rest and collect your thoughts, allow yourself a time of peace and rest every day—or multiple times a day, if necessary—to avoid swings in emotion and to allow for recovery.

Set a pace for yourself that you can keep and do not push yourself too much. If possible, try to take time to rest or take a nap while your baby is sleeping. Trying to do too much can cause setbacks in your health and may affect how well you are able to care for your baby. Many people will want to visit, especially at first, but give yourself the time to take things slowly. Allow others to do things for you if they offer, such as through cooking meals, running errands, or catching up on laundry, in order to give yourself as much time to rest as possible.

The process of delivery puts you at risk of infection, regardless of the type of delivery you had. A vaginal birth may leave you prone to infection if you had any tears or lacerations; you may also have an increased risk of infection if you needed a catheter at any part of the delivery process. If you had a cesarean section, you also face a risk of infection from the surgical site. Your body has already undergone a significant amount of stress and needs time for rest and healing; otherwise, you may be more likely to develop an infection after having your baby.

Another method of reducing your chance of infection is to care for and monitor your incision site if you had one. Follow the directions given to you by your doctor or nurse about how to clean your incision site regularly. You should also try to take a shower each day and wear clean clothes. This will not only keep your body clean, but will support a positive sense of well being. Contact your doctor if you notice any signs of infection and have your blood glucose levels tested during your postpartum visits.

If you develop an infection, you may feel more tired than usual and have pain in the affected area, which is often in the pelvic area, but could also be at the incision site of a cesarean section or episiotomy. You may also develop a fever or have abnormal drainage from the site. An infection after delivery can be very serious, and symptoms should not be ignored. If you do not treat an infection after having a baby, it is possible that it could spread to other parts of the body, including the kidneys or even the bloodstream.

If you had gestational diabetes, you may have experienced a greater number of urinary tract infections because of increased glucose in the urine. The excess glucose attracts bacteria, and too many of a certain type of bacteria can lead to infection. Diabetes also can affect your circulation, particularly if you have poor blood glucose control. If an infection does develop, the body normally sends its defense cells to the site to attack the invading pathogens and to control the infection. These defense mechanisms are sent to the site of infection through the bloodstream. If your circulation is impacted by diabetes, your body may not be able to defend itself as quickly and the infection could get out of control. By taking care of yourself and regulating your blood sugar levels, your body may be more likely to defend itself from infection, which will keep you healthy and strong as you heal after delivery.

WAYS TO REVERSE RISK # 12: ATTEND SUPPORT GROUPS

Many support groups and educational forums are available for women who are pregnant or who have recently delivered babies. These groups can be a source of help and encouragement for mothers, even if they are not directly associated with teaching about diabetes. It is important to reduce stress levels to help control blood glucose levels. Some classes are also available that can provide information and education about type 2 diabetes, weight management, the benefits of exercise, and many other topics that can support and promote healthy lifestyle changes.

TYPES OF CLASSES THAT MAY BE AVAILABLE

Regardless of the state of your health after having your baby, support is essential to get you through the work of caring for your child, the effects of sleep deprivation and schedules, and the stress of raising your child. Some people have great support through family and friends, but no matter whom you lean on for help, you can find advice and encouragement through several different types of support groups.

One good thing about the level of communication available today through the Internet, phones, and messaging systems is that you can find out what groups are available in your community that are supportive to your situation. Even if you live in an area with limited face-to-face meetings, there are still options to "meet" with others online through forums, chat rooms, and video messaging.

Depending on your situation, you may want to seek out other new parents who are managing similar situations as your own. There are groups that offer advice and encouragement for whatever situation you are going through right now, whether it is the best method of feeding your baby, how to get more sleep at night, or whether or not to go back to work. Groups exist that serve specific populations as well, including those of moms with similar racial or ethnic backgrounds, moms with certain religious beliefs, moms who choose certain parenting styles, or moms with every type of living situation.

Take a look around and see what is available for your situation. Decide if or what areas you might need support the most and then look into finding a group that will be encouraging. Avoid any groups that make you feel as if you are making mistakes or are otherwise not doing your best for yourself and your baby. The goal of finding a group to join is to find encouragement and support during this potentially difficult time, and your group should be welcoming and helpful, not closed-off or judgmental.

HOW GROUPS CAN POSITIVELY AFFECT YOUR HEALTH

It may not seem that joining a support group could have much effect on your health and your risk of diabetes after having a baby. However, support groups can positively impact your mental and emotional health, which in turn contributes to positive physical health. Depending on the type of group that you join, you may be inspired to take better care of yourself, increase your physical activity levels, join a gym, volunteer in the community, or any other number of activities that can go a long way toward better health.

Having support from others who are going through the same thing or those who have been through it before can have a significant impact on your stress levels and can positively boost your feelings of well-being. Many groups will also offer education and information about resources available that can help you to take better care of yourself. You may find valuable information from other moms who have successfully managed their health and well being after giving birth and who can share their own tips and tricks.

Some support groups are offered that specifically target a certain situation, such as managing your health after gestational diabetes or preventing type 2 diabetes. These groups might be offered more in the form of classes that are designed to provide education in a learning environment through one or more sessions. These groups are valuable for not only learning important information about how to make lifestyle changes and learning to manage your health, but they can be great places to make new friends and meet other people in similar situations to your own.

Check with your local hospital, school, health care clinic, or community college to see if there are classes available or new groups forming that can provide education about healthy living, breastfeeding, infant care, or managing your blood glucose levels. You can also search online by using search engines or checking links affiliated with whichever topic you are looking for. Some examples of groups that offer support and education during this time include Postpartum Support International, FoodFit, Le Leche League International, or Sidelines National Support Network. The right group can be a wonderful source of support that can reduce feelings of loneliness and isolation, provide new friends and acquaintances, and can help you feel better about your situation. All of these components support stress reduction and positive feelings, which ultimately lead to better health.

WAYS TO REVERSE RISK # 13: CONTROL BLOOD PRESSURE

High blood pressure contributes to diabetes risk as well as further complications after a diabetes diagnosis. Pregnancy can also affect blood pressure levels, which may need continued maintenance, even after the baby is born.

HOW HIGH BLOOD PRESSURE CONTRIBUTES TO DIABETES

Blood pressure is a measurement of the force of blood against the inside of the vessels. It is measured in two numbers: systolic, which is the amount of pressure while the heart contracts; and diastolic, which is the amount of pressure of the blood in between heartbeats. Increased levels of blood pressure can increase your risk of heart attack, stroke, damage to your blood vessels, kidney damage, or eye damage.

High blood pressure also can impact how your body uses insulin, causing increased insulin resistance among the body's cells. The exact relationship of whether high blood pressure causes insulin resistance or whether the reverse relationship is true is still unclear, but there are clear correlations between the two conditions. Regardless of which condition actually causes the other, you can have insulin resistance and high blood pressure at the same time. It is important to monitor and control your blood pressure levels to avoid insulin resistance and resulting uncontrolled blood sugar levels.

Some women develop high blood pressure levels during pregnancy, in a condition that is sometimes referred to as preeclampsia. This dangerous condition typically develops after 20 weeks' gestation and can lead to increased amounts of protein excreted in the urine as well as cause damage to the eyes and brain. It can also affect the placenta, leading to a low birth weight for the baby or the potential for premature birth.

Preeclampsia also affects how your body processes insulin. It increases your risk of later developing type 2 diabetes after you deliver the baby. The Institute for Clinical Evaluative Sciences reported that your risk of developing type 2 diabetes increases two fold if you had preeclampsia during pregnancy. If you had GDM and preeclampsia during pregnancy, your risk jumps to 15 times greater of developing type 2 diabetes over someone who had neither condition.

If you had gestational diabetes during pregnancy, you can reduce your risk of insulin resistance and possibly type 2 diabetes by controlling your blood pressure. Whether or not you had high blood pressure during pregnancy, you should still continue to monitor your blood pressure levels even after you have given birth. You can have your blood pressure checked at your postpartum appointments and many pharmacies or drug stores also have machines that will electronically check your blood pressure, allowing you to monitor your levels and keep tabs on your health.

Ways to Control Blood Pressure after Delivery

There are a number of lifestyle changes that you can implement that will help to control your blood pressure after you've had your baby. It is very important to increase your physical activity and eat a healthy diet, which not only controls your blood pressure levels, but will help to control your weight as well.

A diet called DASH (Dietary Approaches to Stop Hypertension) is useful to help avoid high blood pressure. This diet focuses on whole grains, low-fat dairy, fruits, and vegetables while limiting saturated fat and salt. If you have high blood pressure, you could consider asking your health care provider about the DASH diet. Limiting salt intake is another strategy for managing blood pressure. You can easily reduce the amount of salt you take in by eliminating extra salt added during meal preparation and while eating. Cutting back on processed foods can also reduce your salt intake, as many of these foods are high in sodium.

Other changes that you can make to control your blood pressure include limiting your alcohol intake, and quitting smoking, including regular tobacco smoke use and exposure to secondhand smoke. You can also limit situations that cause stress, as stress and anxiety can cause increased blood pressure, at least on a temporary basis. This is easier said than done, however, as stressful situations may crop up without advance warning. Since it is not possible to eliminate all stress, you can still help your blood pressure by how you deal with stress, such as by taking a time out and taking deep breaths, or taking a short walk to try and clear your head. Caffeine intake also may have an affect on your blood pressure, but the exact reason is not entirely clear.

Even if you are not sure of the effects of caffeine on your blood pressure, you can still positively contribute to your health by cutting back on your caffeine intake. Many caffeinated drinks contain extra sugar and calories, and reducing or eliminating these types of beverages can help your weight, insulin levels, and possibly your blood pressure.

High blood pressure is scary because you may not even know that you have it. Many people with high blood pressure have no symptoms, yet the condition can still cause damage to their circulatory system. Hypertension is classified as a consistent blood pressure reading over 140/90 mmHg, and pre-hypertension is considered as a consistent systolic blood pressure between 120 and 139 mmHg and a consistent diastolic reading between 80 and 90 mmHg. The healthiest measure of blood pressure is to keep both systolic and diastolic pressures at or below 120/80 mmHg. Although it may sound like a daunting task, high blood pressure can be managed well, and many people are able to control their levels relatively easily without using medication. By making the necessary lifestyle changes, high blood pressure does not have to increase your risk for later health problems.

WAYS TO REVERSE RISK # 14: CONSIDER FUTURE PREGNANCIES

For women with GDM, the risk of having diabetes during future pregnancies is increased. Further pregnancies with gestational diabetes increase the lifetime risk of developing type 2 diabetes. Management of blood glucose levels and weight during pregnancy may not only help to manage GDM if it does develop during another pregnancy, but may also reduce the risk of developing type 2 diabetes later in life.

PREGNANCY PLANNING AND CONTRACEPTION

Unfortunately, if you had GDM with your last pregnancy, your risk of having it again is higher if you decide to have another baby. Depending on your situation, thoughts of a future pregnancy may be daunting, especially if you had a difficult time managing your gestational diabetes or if you had a difficult labor or delivery. Alternatively, if your GDM was managed well and you had few complications, thoughts of a future pregnancy might be easier to consider.

Regardless of your situation, pregnancy planning is important if you have had gestational diabetes. Because you may be more likely to develop GDM with future pregnancies, your future risks of developing type 2 diabetes may be impacted as well. Whatever your thoughts are about future pregnancies: whether you want to go on to have more children, you want to wait a while, or you choose not to have anymore children, carefully consider your choices and take steps to stay healthy and take care of yourself in the process.

Pregnancy can be hard on your body, especially if you have GDM. Careful planning and consideration can help to prepare you for a healthy pregnancy and body if you do decide to have another child. You may need to discuss your plans with a health care provider who can assist you with birth control until you feel ready for a pregnancy again. Your body needs time to heal after giving birth and it takes time for your blood glucose levels to return to normal after having GDM. Planning for the next pregnancy may also reduce the chance of an unsuspected pregnancy in which you must quickly take steps to support your health and take care of yourself while managing changes in your body and a growing baby at the same time.

If you are wary about a future pregnancy because of your experience with GDM in the past, talk with your health care provider about your concerns. Find someone who will listen to your points, even if this means changing to a different provider for your next pregnancy. Make sure that you work with someone who will not only support your decisions for your next pregnancy, labor, and delivery, but who will help you to carefully manage your diabetes as well if it develops again.

THE IMPACT OF DIABETES ON FUTURE PREGNANCIES

If you have had GDM in the past, it is important to monitor your health during future pregnancies. While good nutrition and exercise are very important, they do not necessarily prevent the recurrence of GDM with future pregnancies among all women. If you become pregnant again and you previously had gestational diabetes, you may need to monitor your blood sugar more frequently, such as through random blood sugar testing or more than one oral glucose tolerance test (OGTT). Although the OGTT is typically administered around 28 weeks' gestation, your health care provider may decide to administer this test earlier in your next pregnancy to keep an eye on your blood sugar and your body's response to glucose, in case gestational diabetes develops earlier in this pregnancy.

Above all, careful consideration for future pregnancies can make having a healthy child possible. If you work with a health care provider who knows how to manage GDM and you take proper steps to care for yourself, you will improve your chances of a successful subsequent pregnancy and reverse your risks for developing type 2 diabetes in the future.

Recap of the Steps To Reverse Your Risk

1. Breastfeeding reduces your risk possibly by helping you control your weight and blood sugar levels during the post partum period. It may not be the easiest task, but you can get some help in the hospital and after leaving through the lactation consultants most hospitals have. Breastfeeding for 1-3 months has a significant impact on both you and your baby.

2. Monitoring glucose levels after birth of your baby helps control your risk by making sure your levels return to normal. You also might participate in an oral glucose tolerance test again to make sure the blood sugar levels are remaining normal.

3. Controlling your insulin levels reduces your risk as well. Insulin is released in direct response to the amount of carbohydrate you eat and glucose levels in your blood. By watching your diet, you will reduce the amount of insulin that is released into the blood stream, and keep your blood sugar levels low to boot, so you are healthier and may find it easier to lose weight.

4. Performing regular exercise or physical activity will reverse your risks by using calories and allowing your body to absorb glucose into your muscle cells for use. It can strengthen your heart and muscles as well as enable you to feel better doing normal activities.

5. Setting a weight loss goal might seem odd after just giving birth, but you should plan to return to your pre-term weight as soon as possible. And if that weight was a little high (according to your doctor) you should continue using exercise and diet to lose an additional 5-10% of your body weight to lower your risk for diabetes.

6. Taking medications that help with blood sugar control – such as metformin – to keep your blood sugars under control and help you lose the weight you need to. Even if you don't have diabetes but do have impaired glucose tolerance, you might want to consider starting to manage your glucose levels so they stay below the diabetic range.

7. Attending your checkups with your OB makes sure you are healing and returning to a normal lifestyle. He or she can help with questions you might have about your reproductive health, and provide assistance if you need it. Either your OB or your regular doctor will be doing some follow up testing to make sure your diabetes is no longer present.

8. Monitoring your blood cholesterol levels keeps you healthy as well – and every little bit helps. Lowering the bad cholesterol will keep your heart healthy and lower your risk of heart problems in the future. Many people with diabetes find their high cholesterol and high blood sugar levels go hand in hand, so keep it within the normal range.

9. Returning for additional testing as necessary is important. Even after you have the baby and stop seeing the OB doctor, you will need to keep up with your check ups to make sure the blood sugar does not get too high.

10. Managing your stress and treating any depression is key to keeping your body healthy. Stress is a natural part of having a newborn, but managing it takes a bit of practice. Depression can strike at any time, but make sure you are speaking to your doctor about changes in feelings that seem to be overwhelming to you.

11. Healing from the pregnancy and birth takes some time. Allow your body to manage the process by eating a healthy meal and getting help from others. Newborns can be very demanding, so take a moment to figure out a plan for helpers.

12. Checking into local support groups for breastfeeding, new moms or other related topics is helpful. These groups help you to understand you are not alone and that you can do it.

13. Controlling high blood pressure after the birth is yet another way to reduce your risk. Damage to your kidneys and heart happens before you are diagnosed with diabetes, so you can protect those vital organs by controlling your blood pressure.

14. Considering your next pregnancies is important to your health. If you had gestational diabetes with this pregnancy, you have a good chance of having it again in the next. In that case, take precautions early and start eating right before you are tested so you can prevent issues with the pregnancy.

I wish you luck in reversing your risk of developing type 2 diabetes – you can do it with the suggestions in this book. Please take them to heart and do what you can.

And we would really appreciate it if you took a moment and gave us a review in Amazon for this book. Thanks.

Made in United States
Orlando, FL
28 June 2023